Vegan Cookbook for Athletes

Tasty and High Protein Recipes and Meal Plans for Plant-Based Bodybuilding

Frank Smith

Table of Contents

Vegan Diet and Athletes

Getting your body in shape requires figuring out the kind of diet you can hold indefinitely. This would most commonly be a diet that's affordable, light on your digestion, and in line with your personal beliefsand lifestyle.

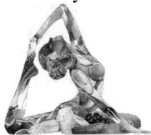

When you add the requirement of achieving athletic results on a vegan diet, you've entered a whole new paradigm of eating that comes down to having a scientifically based and competitive diet that lets you achieve your inner potential to the fullest.

Veganism. You see it all over the place, and lots and lots of people like to talk about it, which, of course, leads to a completely reliable source of information... ha! Wouldn't that be great? But, as humanity kicks in, you start to realize that a lot of these sources are completely untrustworthy.

Now, as more and more people talk about it and more and more opinions get thrown around, mixed in with some fallacies and judgments, combined with some paranoia, and you get yourself a nice, tasty Stew of Ignorance with just a dabble of

truth at the bottom, but you can't even see it because of all the stuff floating around on top of it. Don't drink the Stew of Ignorance! Instead, look for real sources who are on the side of the facts (that's me). Through the new chapters, I'll be taking various things out of the Stew of Ignorance until we get to the root of the matter.

The first "ingredient" that mucks up the Stew of Ignorance is myths. Myths, myths, myths. There's about a bazillion of them associated with veganism, but let's knock off each one, one at a time, good and bad, and

give you a real picture of what veganism is actually about. Pour out that Stew of Ignorance!

Myth Number 1: The biggest one is that veganism cannot actually sustain you. You've probably heard this argument before, maybe even toted with a "we aren't rabbits, you know." Funny? Yes. But also completely untrue. Now, there is some merit to this argument, and here it is: if you don't do it right, cutting out meat and dairy products can lead to some deficiencies (like vitamin B, calcium deficiencies, etc.). Here's the thing it all boils down to: if you don't plan, no diet will really work. Before starting such a diet, make sure to be knowledgeable about the potential drawbacks and plan for them, thus destroying Myth Number 1.

Myth Number 2: Veganism makes you healthier than normal diets! It's the exact opposite of Myth Number 1, and it's also just… well, it's just not entirely correct. Yes, various studies have shown that people who are vegans tend to have lower rates of heart disease and cancers and actually just feel better in general. On face value, hooray! Veganism fixes everything! The truth is a bit more complicated: most people who are vegans also practice very healthy lifestyles and, once you remove the figures about meat-eaters who skew the data with terrible health (cigarette smokers, overeaters, etc.), there's about the same low rate between vegans and non-vegans. So, yes, if you are a healthy person and you take care of yourself, you will be better off both in the short and long term.

Myth Number 3: Veganism leads to protein deficiencies. Essential amino acids, which, you guessed it, are essential, serve as the building blocks that make up protein. The body can't make them all, so you have to eat them. Yes, many plant proteins have a pretty low number of essential amino acids (which is protein, basically), which would be terrible if you only ate these foods. However, this can be easily bypassed through the use of other plant-based proteins, like rice and beans, nuts, seeds, legumes, etc. In other words, make sure you're not just having one kind of thing and watch what you eat, and you should have no problems with protein deficiencies. There are a lot of myths about not veganism making people tired, weak, etc., but it all is this same thing: combine foods to properly dodge this. We'll be including some meal plans at the end.

BREAKFAST

1. Carrots and Raisins Muffins

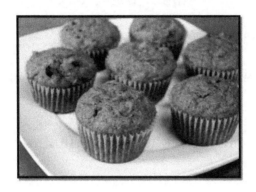

Ready in Time: S5 minutes | Servings: 4

<u>Ingredients</u>

1 1/4 cup almond flour

1/2 cup whole grain flour (any) 3 Tbsp ground almonds

2 cups carrot, grated 1 1/2 tsp baking soda 2 tsp baking powder 2 tsp cinnamon

1/2 tsp salt

1 tsp apple vinegar

1/2 cup extra-virgin olive oil 2 Tbsp linseed oil

4 Tbsp organic honey 3 oz raisins seedless

Instructions

1. Preheat oven to 360 F.

2. In a big bowl, combine together almond flour, whole grain flour, baking soda, baking powder, cinnamon, and salt.

3. In a separate bowl, whisk apple vinegar, olive oil, linseed oil, andhoney.

4. Combine almond flour mixture with liquid mixture; stir well.

5. Add in the shredded carrots and raisins; stir well.

6. Fill the muffin cups 3/4 of the way full.

7. Bake for 30 minutes.

8. Remove from the oven, and allow to cool for 10 minutes.

9. Serve.

Nutrition Facts

Percent daily values based on the Reference Daily Intake (RDI) for a2000 calorie diet.

Amount Per Serving

Calories 352.31 | Calories From Fat (28%) 100.15 | Total Fat 11.51g 18% | Saturated Fat 1.4g 7% | Cholesterol 0mg 0% | Sodium 813.86mg 34% | Potassium 736.68mg 21% | Total Carbohydrates 62.35g 21% | Fiber 5g 20% | Sugar 33.82g | Protein 7.42g 11%

2. Green Protein Tornado Smoothie

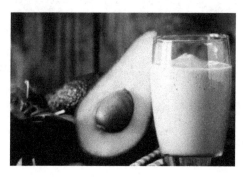

Ready in Time: 10 minutes | Servings:2

Ingredients

1 avocado (diced) 1 cup fresh spinach (chopped)

1 cup fresh peppermint leaves, chopped 1 banana frozen or fresh

1 cup coconut milk canned 1/2 cup shredded coconut

1/2 cup ground nuts (almonds, peanuts) 1 scoop vegan pea protein powder

2 Tbsp extracted honey (or to taste)Ice cubes

Instructions

1. Place all ingredients in your high-speed blender and blend untilsmooth.

2. Serve in chilled glasses with ice cubes.

Nutrition Facts

Percent daily values based on the Reference Daily Intake (RDI) for a2000 calorie diet.

Amount per Serving

Calories 805.81 | Calories From Fat (67%) 542.27 | Total Fat 64.73g 100% | Saturated Fat 32.11g 161% Cholesterol 1.16mg <1% | Sodium 64.66mg 3% | Potassium 1450mg 41% | Total Carbohydrates 53.5g 18% | Fiber 14.19g 57% | Sugar 28.2g | Protein 18.14g 36%

3. **Multi Protein Smoothie**

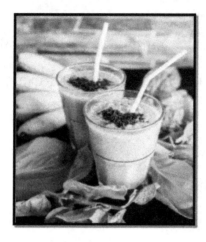

Ready in Time: 10 minutes | Servings:2

Ingredients

2 cups of soy milk

1 scoop soy protein powder4 Tbsp Steel-cut oatmeal

4 Tbsp grated nuts

2 cups fresh spinach, coarsely chopped 1 ripe banana, fresh or frozen 1/2 tsp ground cinnamon 1/2 tsp ground nutmeg 1/2 tsp ground cloves Tbsp Maple syrup or honey 1 tsp pure vanilla extract 2 Tbsp chia seeds for serving

Instructions

1. Combine all the ingredients in your fast-speed blender.

   2. Run the blender until all ingredients are thoroughly blended andsmooth.

3. Sprinkle with chia seeds and serve.

Nutrition Facts

Percent daily values based on the Reference Daily Intake (RDI) for a2000 calorie diet.

Amount Per Serving

Calories 409.84 | Calories From Fat (32%) 131.8 | Total Fat 15.33g 24% |Saturated Fat 1.7g 8% |

Cholesterol 1.16mg <1% | Sodium 187.28mg 8% | Potassium 846,4mg 24% | Total Carbohydrates 55g 18% | Fiber 6.36g 25% |Sugar 35.36g | Protein 16.4g 32%

4. Nutty Silken Tofu with Berries Smoothie

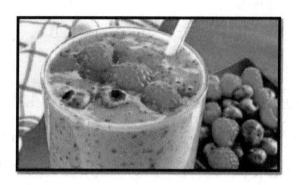

Ready in Time: 10 minutes | Servings:2

Ingredients

1 cup of soy milk 1/2 cup of silken tofu

1   Tbsp almond butter (unsweetened) 1 frozen banana sliced

2   Tbsp Steel-cut oatmeal2 Tbsp ground almonds 2 Tbsp ground cashews 1 tsp pure vanilla extract

1 cup fresh or frozen berries (blueberries, raspberries, blackberries, andstrawberries)

2 Tbsp agave or maple syrup

Instructions

1. Add all ingredients in your high-speed blender.

2. Blend until smooth. Serve and enjoy your liquid

breakfast.

Nutrition Facts

Percent daily values based on the Reference Daily Intake (RDI) for a2000 calorie diet.

Amount Per Serving

Calories 534.45 | Calories From Fat (32%) 173.5 | Total Fat 20.38g 31% |Saturated Fat 2.49g 12% |

Cholesterol 0mg 0% | Sodium 122mg 5% | Potassium 744.56mg21% | Total Carbohydrates 76.7g 26% | Fiber 6.78g 27% | Sugar 35.7g | Protein 17.6g 32%

5. Oat - Raspberries Granola

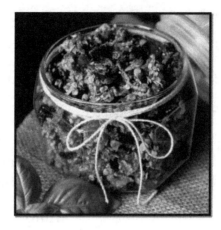

Ready in Time: S5 minutes | Servings: 5

Ingredients

2 cups oats 1/2 cup oat bran

2 Tbsp flaxseed meal

2/3 cup almonds, chopped1/2 cup shredded coconut

1/2 cup dried cranberries, chopped1 tsp cinnamon

1/4 tsp salt Tbsp sesame oil

3 Tbsp maple syrup or honey

1 cup raspberries row or frozen

Instructions

1. Preheat the oven to 325 F/160 C.

2. Stir together the oats, oat bran, flax, almonds, coconut, dried fruit,cinnamon, and salt.

3. In a bowl, stir together sesame oil and maple syrup and microwave forabout 30 seconds.

4. Stir and then microwave for a further 30 seconds.

5. Pour the hot mixture over the dry and stir to combine well.Spread a mixture evenly into a baking tray.

6. Sprinkle fresh raspberries evenly over the mixture

7. Bake for 18-20 minutes.Serve hot or cold with vegetable milk, honey, fruits, etc.

8. Store cold granola an airtight container, in a cool, dry spot for sixmonths (sometimes longer).

Nutrition Facts

Percent daily values based on the Reference Daily Intake (RDI) for a2000 calorie diet.

Amount Per Serving

Calories 590.72 | Calories From Fat (34%) 199.78 | Total Fat 23.85g 37% | Saturated Fat 4.38g 22% | Cholesterol 0mg 0% | Sodium 212.23mg 9% | Potassium 704mg 20% | Total Carbohydrates 81.68g 27% | Fiber 14.2g 60% | Sugar 17.48g | Protein 19g 38%

6. Almond Queen Fruit Smoothie

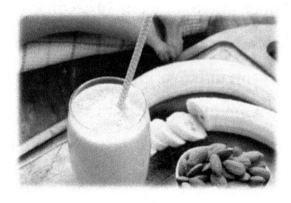

Ready in Time: 10 minutes | Servings: 2

Ingredients

1 1/2 cup almond milk

1 small peeled banana cut into 1-inch chunks and frozen1 cup frozen peaches, sliced, thawed

3 Tbsp toasted almonds ground

1 scoop protein powder (pea or soy)1 Tbsp flaxseed (ground)

Instructions

1. Add all ingredients into a high-speed blender and blend until smooth.

2. Pour your smoothie into the bottle, glass, or Mason jars; cover and keep refrigerated up to 2 days.

3. Or, pour your smoothie into a freezer-safe Ziploc bag and freeze up to3 months.

4. Let it defrost in the refrigerator overnight, stir and enjoy!

Nutrition Facts

Percent daily values based on the Reference Daily Intake (RDI) for a2000 calorie diet.

Amount Per Serving

Calories 262 | Calories From Fat (26%) 67.61 | Total Fat 8g 12% |

Saturated Fat 0.7g 3% | Cholesterol 1.16mg <1% | Sodium 26.49mg 1% | Potassium 497.5mg 14% | Total Carbohydrates 45.27g 15% |

Fiber 5.6g 21% | Sugar 34.85g | Protein 6.58g 13%

7. Baked Raisins & Pumpkin Energy Bars

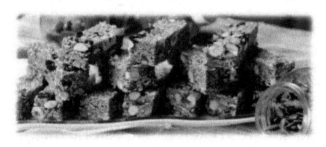

Ready in time: S5 minutes | Servings: 8

Ingredients

1 Tbsp olive oil for greasing 1 tsp pure vanilla extract

1/2 cup of applesauce

1   1/2 cups of rolled oats 2/3 cup golden raisins

1/2 cup of toasted hazelnuts, chopped 1/2 cup of pumpkin seeds

2   tsp vegan protein powder (e.g., chia, soy or hemp) 1/4 tsp cinnamon

1/2 tsp ginger

Pinch of salt to taste

Instructions

1. Preheat the oven to 350 F.

2. Grease a square baking dish.

3. Stir the vanilla extract and applesauce in a large.

4. Stir the oats into the applesauce mixture.

5. Add all remaining ingredients and stir until thoroughly combined.

6. Spoon mixture into the prepared baking dish and press down untileven.

7. Place into oven and bake for about 25 minutes.

8. Remove from the oven, and allow it to cool down completely.

9. Slice into 16 small (or eight large) square or rectangle bars.Wrap each bar with the paper and store at room temperature for up to3 weeks.Also, you can freeze your energy bars in airtight container orfreezer bag to keep it fresh for longer.

Nutrition Facts

Percent daily values based on the Reference Daily Intake (RDI) for a 2000 calorie diet.

Amount Per Serving

Calories 279.13 | Calories From Fat (39%) 109.62 | % Daily Value | Total Fat 12.3g 20% | Saturated Fat 1.24g 6% | Cholesterol 0.19mg <1% | Sodium 303.7mg 13% | Potassium 318.72mg 9% | Total Carbohydrates 38.1g 13% | Fiber 4.16g 17% | Sugar 16.48g | Protein 6g 11%

8. Baked Savory Oat-Apple Bars

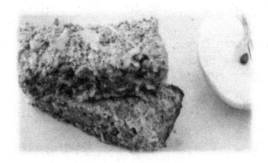

Ready in Time: 45 minutes | Servings: 8

Ingredients

1 Tbs sesame oil (or olive oil)2 tart apples grated

1/2 cup Instant oats 1/2 cup of Rolled oats 1 cup oat flour 1/4 tsp salt tsp baking powder3/4 cup of dates

2/3 cup sesame butter or tahini3 Tbsp Chia seeds

1/2 cup of almond milk 1 tsp pure vanilla extract

Instructions

1. Preheat oven to 350 F.

2. Grease a 9×9" baking pan with oil.

3. Peel and grate apples; place in a colander to drain. In a large bowl, combine Instant and Rolled oats, oat flour, salt, and baking powder. In a separate bowl, stir drained apple, dates, sesame butter, Chia seeds, almond milk, and vanilla extract

until everything is combined well (use a mixer).

4. Add apple mixture to the oat mixture and stir until all ingredients are well incorporated

5. Place the batter into a prepared baking pan.

6. Place in the oven, and bake for 30 minutes.

7. Remove pan from the oven, and let cool completely before slicing. Store bars in a sealed container at room temperature for up to 4 days or refrigerate up to one week.

Nutrition Facts

Percent daily values based on the Reference Daily Intake (RDI) for a 2000 calorie diet.

Amount Per Serving

Calories 316 | Calories From Fat (41%) 130.2 | Total Fat 15.8g 24% | Saturated Fat 2.1g 11% | Cholesterol 0mg 0% | Sodium 208mg 9% | Potassium 353.85mg 10% | Total Carbohydrates 41.74g 14% | Fiber 7.16g 29% | Sugar 16g | Protein 7.62g 15%

9. **Boosting** **Celery-Coconut** **Smoothie**

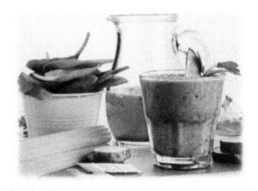

Ready in Time: 10 minutes | Servings: 2

Ingredients

1 celery stalks, chopped

2   cup kale leaves, fresh and chopped 1 large banana cut into slices 1 1/2 cup coconut milk (canned)

1 Tbsp protein powder (pea or soy) 1 Tbsp lemon juice

1 Tbsp chia seeds

Instructions

1. Add all ingredients in your blender and blend until smooth. Pour your smoothie into the bottle, glass, or Mason jars; cover and keep refrigerated up to 2 days. Or, pour your smoothie into a freezer-

safe Ziploc bag and freeze up to 3 months.Let it defrost in the refrigerator overnight, stir and enjoy!Nutrition FactsPercent daily values based on the Reference Daily Intake (RDI) for a 2000 calorie diet.

Amount Per Serving

Calories 473.21 | Calories From Fat (70%) 333.57 | Total Fat 39.7g 61% |Saturated Fat 32.49g 162% | Cholesterol 1.16mg <1% | Sodium 89mg 4% | Potassium 926.64mg 26% | Total Carbohydrates 28.8g 10% | Fiber 6.1g 24% | Sugar 9.5g | Protein 9.2g 18%

10.   **Breakfast Potato Patties**

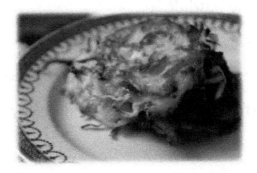

Ready in Time: 45 minutes Servings: 8

Ingredients

1 1/2 lb grated potatoes1 grated onion

3 Tbsp applesauce unsweetened (canned) Salt and ground black pepper to taste

2 Tbsp all-purpose flour

1/2 cup olive or canola oil for frying

Instructions

1. Add all ingredients In a large bowl, and stir until all ingredientscombined well.

2. Form the batter into flat patties.

3. Heat oil in a large frying skillet over medium heat.

4. Fry your potato patties for about 6 to 7

minutes, and then flip with a spatula and fry from the other side until done.

5. Remove ready patties on a plate lined with kitchen paper to drain, andcompletely cool.

6. Transfer your patties in a single layer to baking sheets.

7. Freeze patties until hard.

8. Transfer the frozen patties to freezer bags and keep in freeze up to 2weeks.

9. Reheat in a microwave oven.

Nutrition Facts

Percent daily values based on the Reference Daily Intake (RDI) for a2000 calorie diet.

Amount Per Serving

Calories 201.55 | Calories From Fat (60%) 121.42 | Total Fat 13.74g 21% | Saturated Fat 1g 5% | Cholesterol 0mg 0% | Sodium 5.87mg <1% | Potassium 386.69mg 11% | Total Carbohydrates 18.2g 6% | Fiber 2.25g 9%| Sugar 1.5g | Protein 2.8g 6%

LUNCH

11. Asian Chilled Cucumber and Seaweed Soup

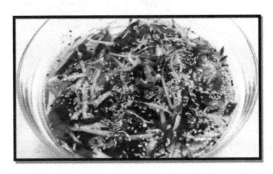

Ready in Time: 15 minutes | Servings: 6

Ingredients

1 cup soaked seaweed, rinsed * see note 2 cucumbers cut into thin slices Seasonings

4 Tbsp of soy sauce

1/4 cup fresh lemon juice 1/2 tsp garlic minced

1 Tbsp red pepper flakes 2 tsp sesame seeds toasted 1 tsp brown sugar

4 cups of water Sea salt to taste

Instructions

1. Soak seaweed in water to cover overnight.

2. When soft, drain and cut into 2-inch pieces.

3. Boil water with a little salt in a pot.

4. Blanch drained seaweed for 20 to 25 seconds; plunge into the icewater.

5. In a bowl, combine together cucumber, seaweed, and all remainingingredients; stir well.

6. Refrigerate to chill well.

7. Taste and adjust salt to taste.

8. Serve in chilled bowls.

Nutrition Facts

Percent daily values based on the Reference Daily Intake (RDI) for a2000 calorie diet.

Amount Per Serving

Calories 49.06 | Calories From Fat (15%) 7.18 | Total Fat 0.86g 1%

| Saturated Fat 0.2g 1% | Cholesterol 0mg 0% | Sodium 440.87mg 18%

| Potassium 238,19mg 7% | Total Carbohydrates 10.11g 3% | Fiber1.29g 5% | Sugar 3.41g | Protein 3g 6%

Note: **Because of its increasing popularity, many major supermarket chains carry dried seaweed in their Asian foods aisle.**

12.   Baked "Hasselback" Sweet Potatoes

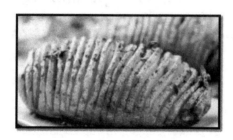

Ready in Time: 1 hour and 15 minutes | Servings: 4

Ingredients

1/2 cup olive oil Tbsp of fresh rosemary finely chopped 4 large sweet potatoes, chopped 1/2 tsp ground mustard Kosher salt and freshly ground black pepper1 cup Tofu grated (optional)

Instructions

1. Preheat oven to 425 F.

2. Wash and rub potatoes; cut trough potatoes about halfway into thin slices (as Hasselback potatoes).Combine olive, rosemary, and ground mustard; generously brush potatoes.Place sweet potatoes on a greased baking sheet.Bake for 60

minutes or until soft.Remove from the oven, and let cool for 10 minutes.Serve with grated Tofu (optional).

Nutrition Facts

Percent daily values based on the Reference Daily Intake (RDI) for a2000 calorie diet.

Amount Per Serving

Calories 285.21 | Calories From Fat (92%) 263.44 | Total Fat 30g 46% |Saturated Fat 4g 20% |Cholesterol 0mg 0% | Sodium 12.48mg <1% | Potassium 69.92mg2% | Total Carbohydrates 1.13g <1% | Sugar 0.25g | Protein 5g 10%

13. Baked Buffalo Cauliflower 'Wings

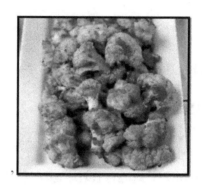

Ready in Time: S0 minutes | Servings: 4

Ingredients

1   Tbsp olive oil1 cup of soy milk1 cup soy flour

2 tsp garlic powder 1 head of cauliflower, chopped into flowerets 1 cup Red Hot Sauce (or vegan Buffalo sauce) 2 Tbsp of avocado oil

Instructions

1. Preheat the oven to 450 F/225 C.

2. Grease a shallow baking dish with olive oil; set aside.

3.   In a bowl, stir together soy milk, soy flour, and garlic powderuntil well combined.

4. Coat the cauliflower florets with the soy flour

mixture and place in aprepared baking dish.

5. Bake for 18 to 20 minutes.

6. In a meanwhile, heat Red Hot Sauce or vegan Buffalo sauce withavocado oil in a saucepan.

7. Pour the hot sauce over the baked cauliflower and bake for anadditional 6 to 8 minutes.

8. Serve hot.

Nutrition Facts

Percent daily values based on the Reference Daily Intake (RDI) for a2000 calorie diet.

Amount Per Serving

Calories 360.35 | Calories From Fat (63%) 225.7 | Total Fat 25.93g 40% |Saturated Fat 3.54g 18% |

Cholesterol 0mg 0% | Sodium 953.78mg 40% | Potassium 1286.29mg 37% | Total Carbohydrates 23.49g 8% | Fiber 7.32g 29% | Sugar 8g | Protein 14g 28%

14.   Baked Creamy Corn with Shredded Tofu

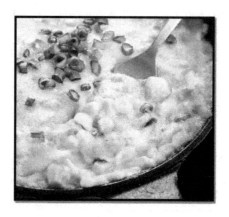

Ready in Time: 25 minutes | Servings: 4

Ingredients

4 Tbsp rice oil

3 cups sweet corn kernels (frozen or fresh) 2 green onions, thinly sliced

1 cup vegan mayonnaise 1 Tbsp brown sugar

Salt and pepper to taste 8 oz silken tofu shredded

Instructions

1. Preheat oven to 400 F/200 C.

2. Grease a baking dish with rice oil.

3.   In a bowl, combine together corn kernels, green onions. Vegan mayonnaise, brown sugar, and salt and pepper; stir to combine well.

4. Pour the corn mixture into a prepared baking dish.

5. Sprinkle evenly with shredded tofu.

6. Bake for 14 to 16 minutes.

7. Remove from the oven and allow it to cool.

8. Serve.

Nutrition Facts

Percent daily values based on the Reference Daily Intake (RDI) for a2000 calorie diet.

Amount Per Serving

Calories 482 | Calories From Fat (65%) 312.49 | Total Fat 35.37g 54% |Saturated Fat 5.86g 29% |

Cholesterol 15.28mg 5% | Sodium 425.49mg 18% | Potassium 338.68mg 10% | Total Carbohydrates 40.56g 14% | Fiber 2.4g 10% | Sugar 10.48g | Protein 7.16g 14%

15. Baked Tamari-Tofu and Cabbage Salad

Ready in Time: 45 minutes | Servings: 4

Ingredients

1 lb firm tofu, drained and cut into 1/2-inch slabs1/2 cup tamari sauce

1 lb shredded cabbage2 shredded carrots

1 onion finely sliced

Sea salt and ground pepper to taste4 Tbsp sesame oil

1 Tbsp fresh ginger grated1 tsp hot chili paste

3 Tbsp rice vinegar or apple cider vinegar2 cloves garlic minced Tbsp water

Instructions

1. Preheat the oven to 375 degrees F.

2. Grease a baking sheet with some oil and set aside.

3. Toss Tofu slabs with 1/4 cup of the tamari sauce.

4. Arrange the tofu on the prepared baking sheet and bake for 25 to 30minutes.

5. Remove from the oven and set aside to cool.

6.   In a large bowl, combine the cabbage, carrots, and onion; season with the salt and pepper, and set aside.

7.   In a separate bowl, combine sesame oil, ginger, chili paste, and remaining 1/4 cup of tamari sauce, vinegar, garlic, and water.

8. Pour the garlic-ginger mixture over the cabbage mixture and toss to combine.

9. Taste and adjust seasonings. Serve topped with tofu.

Nutrition Facts

Percent daily values based on the Reference Daily Intake (RDI) for a 2000 calorie diet.

Amount Per Serving

Calories 386 | Calories From Fat (55%) 213.87 | Total Fat 24.8g 38% | Saturated Fat 3.58g 18% | Cholesterol 0mg 0% | Sodium 2080mg 87% | Potassium 759.94mg 22% | Total Carbohydrates 21.52g 7% | Fiber 7.1g 31% | Sugar 7.54g | Protein 25.8g 52%

16. Aromatic Spinach with Basil-Sesame Puree

Ready in Time: S0 minutes | Servings: 4

Ingredients

1 lb fresh spinach 4 Tbsp of olive oil

1 onion finely chopped 1 leek finely chopped 3 cloves

garlic 3 cup of vegetable broth 4 Tbsp grated tomato

1 cup fresh basil finely chopped 1/3 cup sesame oil

Salt and ground pepper to taste

Instructions

1. Boil spinach in salted water for 3 to 5 minutes.
2. Remove from heat and place in colander to drain.
3. Heat oil in a frying skillet over medium-high heat. Sauté the onion, leek, and garlic with a pinch of salt, often stirring, for about 5 to 6 minutes.
4. Pour vegetable broth, grated tomato, and basil leaves; stir for 2 minutes. Add spinach, give a good stir, cover, and cook for 6 - 8 minutes over medium-low heat. Transfer the spinach mixture in a blender, and

add the sesame oil; blend for 30 seconds or until smooth. Taste and adjust salt and pepper.

5. Store in an airtight container and freeze for a month.

Nutrition Facts

Percent daily values based on the Reference Daily Intake (RDI) for a 2000 calorie diet.

Amount Per Serving

Calories 381.85 | Calories From Fat (77%) 295.2 | Total Fat 33.53g 52% | Saturated Fat 4.68g 23% | Cholesterol 0.46mg <1% | Sodium 843.36mg 35% | Potassium 552.58mg 16% | Total Carbohydrates 17.7g 6% | Fiber 6g 24% | Sugar 3.14g | Protein 6.76g 14%

17. Baked Quinoa and Black Beans Patties

Ready in Time: 1 hour and 5 minutes | Servings: 2

Ingredients

1 cup of quinoa1 cup of water

1 can (15 oz) of black beans4 Tbsp sesame seeds

4 Tbsp bread crumbs2 Tbsp tomato paste

1 Tbsp hot sauce (any) 2 Tbsp nutritional yeast1 tsp garlic powder

1/2 tsp of oregano 1/2 tsp of rosemary

1 Tbsp fresh basil finely chopped Salt and ground black pepper to taste**Instructions**

1. In a pot, cook quinoa for about 15 minutes.

2. Place in a colander, and drain; let quinoa to cool down.

3. Preheat oven to 400 F.

4. Line a baking sheet with baking paper.

5. In a bowl, add black beans and mash with a fork.

6. Add quinoa, sesame seeds, and all remaining ingredients; stir untilcombine well.

7. Roll dough into balls.

8. Place quinoa balls/patties on a prepared baking sheet.

9. Bake for about 35 minutes.

10. Remove from the oven, and allow to cool completely.

11.   Store in an airtight container and keep refrigerated up to 4 to 5 days. Yield: 4 large patties

Nutrition Facts

Percent daily values based on the Reference Daily Intake (RDI) for a 2000 calorie diet.

Amount Per Serving

Calories 614,39 | Calories From Fat (21%) 130,31 | Total Fat 15.29g 24%

| Saturated Fat 2.51g 13% | Cholesterol 0.21mg <1% | Sodium 719.14mg 30% | Potassium 1312.62mg 39% | Total Carbohydrates 93.57g 31% | Fiber 25g 100% | Sugar 5.48g | Protein 32g 64%

18.   **Barley and Broccoli Pilaf**

Ready in Time: 55 minutes | Servings: 4

Ingredients

. 4 Tbsp olive oil 1 onion, chopped

salt and fresh ground pepper to taste 1 cup pearled barley

2 cups of vegan vegetable broth1 cup of water

1 tsp fresh thyme

1 1/2 cup broccoli florets, cut into small pieces 1/4 cup green peas

1   carrot finely sliced1 tomato sliced

Instructions

1. Heat oil in a large frying pan; sauté onion with a pinch of salt for 2 to 3minutes.

2. Add barley and constantly stir for a further 2 minutes.

3. Add vegetable broth, thyme, and water and bring to boil.

4. Cover, reduce heat to low and simmer for 30 minutes.

5. Add all remaining ingredients, stir well, and

cook for further 20minutes.

6. Taste and adjust the salt and pepper to taste.

7. Allow it to cool completely.

8. Store barley pilaf in an airtight container and keep refrigerated up to 5days.

9. Or, place in freezer bags and keep in the freezer for one month.

Nutrition Facts

Percent daily values based on the Reference Daily Intake (RDI) for a2000 calorie diet.

Amount Per Serving

Calories 409.46 | Calories From Fat (37%) 151.2 | Total Fat 17.15g 26% | Saturated Fat 2.51g 13% | Cholesterol 0.62mg <1% | Sodium 635.47mg 26% | Potassium 588.46mg 17% | Total Carbohydrates 58.38g 19% | Fiber 11.61g 46% | Sugar 5.36g | Protein 8.63g 17%

19.   Cabbage and Cauliflower Puree

Ready in Time: S0 minutes | Servings: 4

Ingredients

water for cooking

1/2 medium head cabbage 1/2 lb cauliflower florets 1 leek finely sliced

2   stalks fresh celery chopped4 Tbsp olive oil

Salt and pepper to taste

Instructions

1. Heat water (about 4 1/2 cups) in a big pot and add all vegetables andoil; season with the little salt.

2. Bring to boil, reduce heat to medium, cover, and cook for about 15 -20minutes.

3. Transfer vegetables in a blender; blend until smooth and combinedwell.

4. Taste and adjust the salt and pepper to taste.

5. Store in an airtight container and keep refrigerated up to 3 to 4 days.

Nutrition Facts

Percent daily values based on the Reference Daily Intake (RDI) for a 2000 calorie diet.

Amount Per Serving

Calories 176.15 | Calories From Fat (69%) 122.33 | Total Fat 13.85g 21%

| Saturated Fat 2g 10% | Cholesterol 0mg 0% | Sodium 43.22mg 2% | Potassium 413.19mg 12% | Total Carbohydrates 12.7g 4% | Fiber 4.43g 18% | Sugar 5.6g | Protein 3g 6%

20. **Dark Red Vegan Soup**

Ready in Time: 1 hour and 10 minutes | Servings: 4

<u>Ingredients</u>

4 Tbsp olive oil

1 onion finely diced

2 cloves garlic finely chopped

salt and freshly ground black pepper 1 lb tomatoes, peeled and grated

2 beets, large, peeled and cut into pieces 2 carrots cut into strips

3/4 tsp cumin

1 tsp cayenne pepper

4 cups of vegetable broth

<u>Instructions</u>

1. Heat the oil in a large pot on medium-high temperature.

    2. Add the onion and garlic and sauté with the pinch of salt, oftenstirring, for about 3 to 4 minutes.

3. Add grated tomatoes, beets, and carrots, and stir for 2 to 3 minutes.

4. Add all remaining ingredients and stir well.

5. Reduce heat to medium-low, cover, and cook for about 50 to 60minutes.

6. Remove from heat; taste and adjust the salt and pepper to taste.

7. Allow to cool down and store in an airtight container; keep refrigeratedup to 5 days.

Nutrition Facts

Percent daily values based on the Reference Daily Intake (RDI) for a2000 calorie diet.

Amount Per Serving

Calories 162.24 | Calories From Fat (15%) 23.79 | Total Fat 2.69g 4% | Saturated Fat 0.58g 3% | Cholesterol 1.38mg <1% | Sodium 982.38mg 41% | Potassium 808.6mg 23% | Total Carbohydrates 30.6g 10% | Fiber 6g 24% |Sugar 9g | Protein 6g 12%

DINNER

21. Beans and Button Mushrooms "Stew"

Ready in Time: S5 minutes | Servings: 6

Ingredients

4 Tbsp olive oil

1 cup chopped onion1 tsp minced garlic

1 lb fresh button mushrooms, sliced 3/4 tsp dried thyme, crushed

1 tsp red paprika

2 cups vegetable broth

1 can (11 oz) tomatoes crushed

2 can (15 oz) white beans, drained Salt and ground black pepper to taste

Instructions

1. Heat olive oil in a pot over medium-high heat.

2. Add onion, garlic, mushrooms, thyme, and red paprika; sauté forabout 4 to 5 minutes.

3. Pour the vegetable broth and tomatoes, and bring to a boil.

4. Reduce heat to medium, cover and cook for 15 to 17 minutes

5. Add the beans and stir; cook for a further 2 to 3 minutes.

6. Remove from heat and adjust the salt and pepper to taste.

7. Serve warm.

Nutrition Facts

Percent daily values based on the Reference Daily Intake (RDI) for a 2000 calorie diet.

Amount Per Serving

Calories 347.87 | Calories From Fat (27%) 95.33 | Total Fat 10.82g 17% |Saturated Fat 1.65g 8% |

Cholesterol 0.62mg <1% | Sodium 524.34mg 22% | Potassium 1221.5mg 35% | Total Carbohydrates 49g 16% | Fiber 10.43g 42% | Sugar 4.77g | Protein 16.5g 33%

22. Boosting Black Beans and Avocado Salad

Ready in Time: 15 minutes | Servings: 4

Ingredients

2 can (11 oz) black beans drained1 avocado cored, cut into cubes

3/4 cup green onions finely chopped 1 cup corn kernels, drained

1 tomato sliced

1 clove garlic finely sliced

1   red bell pepper cut in strips1 pear cut into cubes

1/2 cup olive oil

1/3 cup fresh lime juice

1/4 tsp salt and ground black pepper to taste 1/2 cup chopped cilantro fresh

2 Tbsp parsley finely chopped

Instructions

1.   In a large and deep bowl combine together black beans, avocado, green onion, corn,

tomato, garlic, pear, and bell pepper.

2. In a separate bowl, combine all remaining ingredients and pour overblack bean mixture.

3. Toss to combine well.

4. Taste and adjust salt and pepper to taste.

5. Serve immediately.

Nutrition Facts

Percent daily values based on the Reference Daily Intake (RDI) for a2000 calorie diet.

Amount Per Serving

Calories 561.44 | Calories From Fat (54%) 305.11 | Total Fat 34.91g 54%

| Saturated Fat 4.87g 24% |

Cholesterol 0mg 0% | Sodium 542mg 23% | Potassium 1072.47mg 31% | Total Carbohydrates 54.76g 18% | Fiber 17.1g 71% | Sugar 9.3g | Protein 13.88g 28%

23. **Brown Rice Pasta Salad with Apple Juice Sauce**

Ready in Time: 15 minutes | Servings: 4

Ingredients

1 lb Brown rice pasta

1 can (11 oz) corn boiled, drained 1/2 cup chopped red onion

1 cup carrots, shredded

2 roasted red peppers cut into slices or cubes 2 cups mushrooms, sliced

1/2 cup olive oil

1/2 cup apple juice canned or bottled 1/3 cup chopped fresh basil

Salt and freshly ground black pepper

Instructions

1. Prepare pasta according to package directions.
2. Drain pasta and rinse with cold water.
3. Add brown rice pasta into a large salad bowl together with corn, red onion, carrot, peppers,

and mushrooms.

4. In a separate bowl, whisk together olive oil, apple juice, basil, and saltand pepper.

5. Pour olive oil sauce over the pasta salad; toss to combine well.

6. Taste and adjust the salt and pepper to taste.

7. Serve or keep refrigerated.

Nutrition Facts

Percent daily values based on the Reference Daily Intake (RDI) for a 2000 calorie diet.

Amount Per Serving

Calories 745.1 | Calories From Fat (33%) 247.48 | Total Fat 28g 43% | Saturated Fat 4g 20% |

Cholesterol 0mg 0% | Sodium 185.64mg 8% | Potassium 517.75mg 15% | Total Carbohydrates 105.67g 35% | Fiber 9.16g 37% | Sugar 6.4g | Protein 19g 38%

24.   **Garlic -Potato Puree**

Ready in Time: S5 minutes | Servings: 6

Ingredients

6 potatoes peeled and halvedWater for cooking

8 cloves of garlic, cleaned3/4 cup olive oil

2 Tbsp white wine vinegar

Kosher salt and ground white pepper

2 Tbsp fresh parsley chopped for serving

Instructions

1. Peel, cut into halves and rinse potatoes.

2. Cook potatoes in boiling water until tender or about 20 to 25minutes for halved potatoes.

3. Transfer potatoes in a colander and drain well.

4. Add garlic and olive oil, some salt and pepper in a high-speedblender; blend until combined.

5. Add potatoes and continue to blend until well combined.

6. Remove mixture to a bowl, pour the vinegar and stir with a spoon.

7. Taste and adjust salt and pepper to taste.

8. Sprinkle with chopped parsley and serve!

9. Keep refrigerated.

Nutrition Facts

Percent daily values based on the Reference Daily Intake (RDI) for a2000 calorie diet.

Amount Per Serving

Calories 413.34 | Calories From Fat (58%) 240.45 | Total Fat 27.21g 42%

| Saturated Fat 3.79g 19% |

Cholesterol 0mg 0% | Sodium 15.23mg <1% | Potassium 919mg 26% | Total Carbohydrates 39.44g 13% | Fiber 4.77g 19% | Sugar 2.5g

| Protein 5g 10%

25.   High Protein Soybean Pasta with Basil

Ready in Time: S5 minutes | Servings: 4

Ingredients

1/2 lb soybean pasta

1 can (11 oz) white bean cooked4 tsp olive oil

4 tsp garlic finely chopped

1 can (15 oz) tomato crushed

1 can (11 oz) tomato paste2 tsp dried oregano

Salt and ground black pepper to taste 1/2 cup fresh basil chopped

Instructions

1. Prepare soybean pasta according to package directions; drain.

2. Mash white beans in a blender; set aside.

3. Heat the oil in a saucepan over medium-high heat.

4. Sauté garlic until soft (do not burn it).

5. Add crushed tomatoes and beans, tomato paste, oregano, salt, andpepper.

6. Bring the sauce to a boil, reduce heat to medium-low, and simmer thesauce for 20 minutes.

7. Remove the sauce from the heat and stir in chopped basil.

8. Pour sauce over pasta and serve.

Nutrition Facts

Percent daily values based on the Reference Daily Intake (RDI) for a 2000 calorie diet.

Amount Per Serving

Calories 564.35 | Calories From Fat (10%) 56.26 | Total Fat 6.44g 10% | Saturated Fat 1.04g 5% |

Cholesterol 0mg 0% | Sodium 766mg 32% | Potassium 1448mg 38% | Total Carbohydrates 102.47g 34% | Fiber 17.64g 71% | Sugar 11.83g | Protein 29g 58%

26. Artichoke Hearths with Brown Rice

Preparation Time: 40 minutes | Servings: 4

Ingredients

1 cup of avocado oil (or sesame oil)

10 canned artichoke hearts, drained and chopped 1 cup cauliflower (divided into florets)

1 cup of brown rice

3 cups of vegetable broth

2 Tbsp of fresh parsley finely chopped 2 Tbsp fresh dill finely chopped

2 Tbsp lemon juice freshly squeezed salt and ground pepper to taste

Instructions

1. Heat oil in a large pot over medium-high heat.
2. Add artichoke hearts and sauté for 5 minutes.
3. Add the cauliflower and sprinkle with the pinch of the salt and pepper; stir for two minutes.
4. Add all remaining ingredients and give a good stir.
5. Bring to a boil and reduce heat to medium.

6. Cover and cook for 25 minutes.

7. Taste and adjust seasonings.

8. Allow to cool down completely.

9. Store in a large airtight container and keep refrigerated up to 4 to 5 days.

10. To reheat, place the rice and artichokes into a heatproof dish and add little water or broth; cover and microwave on HIGH for approximately 1 to 2 minutes.

Nutrition Facts

Percent daily values based on the Reference Daily Intake (RDI) for a2000 calorie diet.

Amount Per Serving

Calories 581.35 | Calories From Fat (45%) 263.17 | Total Fat 29.81g 46%

| Saturated Fat 3.69g 18% | Cholesterol 1.23mg <1% | Sodium 1056mg 44%

| Potassium 932.39mg 27% | Total Carbohydrates 72.6g 24% | Fiber 11.35g 45% | Sugar 0.69g | Protein 12.69g 25%

27. Baked Sweet Potato with Green Beans

Ready in Time: 1 hour and 10 minutes | Servings: 5

Ingredients

2 lbs sweet potatoes cut into cubes 1 tsp pumpkin pie spice

1/3 cup olive oil

3/4 lb canned green beans, drained 1 cup mushrooms (chopped fine) 1 1/2 cups of water

Salt and ground black pepper to taste

Instructions

1. Preheat oven to 350 F.

2. Grease 9-inch baking dish; set aside.

3. Blend the sweet potato cubes, oil, and pumpkin pie spice in a

4. Cover and let it sit for about 5 minutes or until smooth.

5. Arrange the sweet potato mixture over the prepared baking dish, and cover with the green beans mixture.

6. Bake for about 1 hour or until sweet potato is soft.

7. Adjust seasonings and allow to cool completely.

8. Store in an airtight container and keep refrigerated up to 4 days.

Nutrition Facts

Percent daily values based on the Reference Daily Intake (RDI) for a2000 calorie diet.

Amount Per Serving

Calories 158.78 | Calories From Fat (82%) 129.44 | Total Fat 14.65g 23% | Saturated Fat 2g 10% | Cholesterol 0mg 0% | Sodium 6.19mg <1% | Potassium 192.27mg 5% | Total Carbohydrates 6g 2% | Fiber 2.04g 8% | Sugar 2g | Protein 1.64g 3%

28. **Beans and Cauliflower Soup**

Ready in Time: 25 minutes | Servings: 6

<u>Ingredients</u>

1/4 cup olive oil

1 large onion cut in chunks

2 cloves garlic finely chopped salt and ground pepper, to taste2 can (11 oz) white beans

2 cups cauliflower

2 Tbsp chopped parsley3 sprigs thyme

pepper

3 1/2 cups vegetable broth

<u>Instructions</u>

1. Heat oil in a large pot over medium-high heat.

2. Sauté the onion and garlic with a pinch of salt until soft andtranslucent.

3. Add white beans and stir for two minutes.

4. Add cauliflower and stir for one minute.

5. Add all remaining ingredients and stir for one minute.

6. Reduce heat to medium, cover, and cook for 10 minutes.

7. Remove the bean soup in a blender; blend until smooth.

8. Store in an airtight container in the fridge up to 5 days or freeze up to two months.

Nutrition Facts

Percent daily values based on the Reference Daily Intake (RDI) for a 2000 calorie diet.

Amount Per Serving

Calories 463.8 | Calories From Fat (23%) 107.56 | Total Fat 12.19g 19% | Saturated Fat 2g 10% | Cholesterol 2.88mg <1% | Sodium 637.61mg 27% | Potassium 1941mg 55% | Total Carbohydrates 66.48g 22% | Fiber 15.16g 61% | Sugar 3.47g | Protein 25.43g 51%

29. Beans, Sesame and Pine Nuts Puree

Ready in Time: 20 minutes | Servings: 4

Ingredients

1 lb broad beans

2 cups boiling water

salt and ground black pepper to taste 1/3 cup sesame or avocado oil

1 tsp garlic powder

1/4 cup roasted pine nuts 1 Tbsp sesame seeds

1 Tbsp lemon juice, freshly squeezed

Instructions

1. Boil beans in a large pot for 2 minutes, throw water, and rinse them.

    2. Add fresh water, a little salt, and boil broad beans for about 7 to 8minutes.

    3. Transfer broad beans into a high-speed blender along with all remaining ingredients blend until soft.

4. Taste and adjust seasonings.

5. Store in an airtight container and ref up to 5 days.

Nutrition Facts

Percent daily values based on the Reference Daily Intake (RDI) for a2000 calorie diet.

Amount Per Serving

Calories 323.6 | Calories From Fat (66%) 214.7 | Total Fat 24.64g 38% | Saturated Fat 3.04g 15% | Cholesterol 0mg 0% | Sodium 106.16mg 4% | Potassium 458.62mg 13% | Total Carbohydrates 23.15g 8% | Fiber 0.52g 2% | Sugar 0.73g | Protein 10.38g 21%

30. Stuffed Bell Peppers with Rice and Pine Nuts

Ready in Time: 1 hour and 50 minutes | Servings: 8

Ingredients

8 bell peppers (green or red)1 cup of olive oil

1 large onion finely diced3 cloves garlic minced

1 large carrot grated1 cup of rice

1 cup of fresh tomato juice3 Tbsp semolina flour

Salt and ground pepper to taste

2 Tbsp fresh parsley finely chopped 1 Tbsp fresh basil finely chopped

1 cup pine nuts1 cup raisins

juice of 2 tomatoes

Instructions

1. Cut the stems of papers and set aside.

2. Remove seeds from peppers and rinse well; set aside to drain.

3. Heat the half of oil in a large frying skillet and sauté the onion, garlic,rice, carrot on high heat.

4. Reduce the heat to moderate, add the tomato,

semolina, and the salt and pepper; stir well and remove the pan from the heat.

5. Add the herbs, pine nuts, raisins to the mixture, and stir well.

6. Taste and adjust the salt and ground pepper to taste.

7. Preheat oven to 400 F.

8. Fill the peppers with the rice mixture and cover with their stems ortomato slices.

9. Place stuffed peppers into an oiled baking dish and pour with remaining olive oil and some tomato juice.

10. Bake for about 55 to 60 minutes.

11. Remove from the oven, and let it sit until cool completely.

12. Keep refrigerated in one or two airtight containers up to 4 to 5 days or freeze for up to a month.

Nutrition Facts

Percent daily values based on the Reference

Daily Intake (RDI) for a2000 calorie diet.

Amount Per Serving

Calories 426.48 | Calories From Fat (56%) 238.7 | Total Fat 27.38g 42% | Saturated Fat 3.29g 16% | Cholesterol 0mg 0% | Sodium 93mg 4% | Potassium 605.08mg 17% | Total Carbohydrates 43.86g 15% | Fiber 6.81g 27% | Sugar 12.55g | Protein 5.86g 12%

31. Sweet Red and Black Chili with Cinnamon

Ready in Time: 45 minutes | Servings: 6

Ingredients

4 Tbs of olive oil onion finely diced

1 cloves garlic, chopped 1 red pepper cut into small cubes

Kosher salt and ground black pepper to taste 1 can (15 oz) red beans, cooked 1 can (11 oz) of black beans can (11 oz) crushed tomatoes 2 tsp chili powder 1/4 tsp ground cinnamon

1 Tbsp fresh parsley finely chopped 2 cups of vegetable broth

Instructions

1. Press the SAUTÉ button on your Instant Pot.

2. When the word "hot" appears on display, add the oil and sauté the onion and garlic with a pinch of salt and pepper until soft; stir occasionally.

3. Add red pepper and stir for one minute.

4. Add red and black beans and stir for one minute.

5. Add all remaining ingredients and give a good stir. Lock lid into place and set on the MANUAL setting high pressure for20 minutes.

6. When the beep sounds, use the Natural pressure release for 15 minutes. Taste and adjust salt and pepper to taste. Store in an airtight container in the fridge for up to 5 days.

7. Or, let the chili cool a bit, then pack it in a freezer bag or Tupperware container and keep in freezer up to 3 months.

Nutrition Facts

Percent daily values based on the Reference Daily Intake (RDI) for a 2000 calorie diet.

Amount Per Serving

Calories 266.41 | Calories From Fat (34%) 90.97 | Total Fat 10.39g 16% | Saturated Fat 1.58g 8% | Cholesterol 0mg 0% | Sodium 464.62mg 19% | Potassium 686.1mg 20% | Total Carbohydrates 33.73g 11% | Fiber 11.23g 45% | Sugar 4.84g | Protein 12.1g 24%

SNACKS

32. Beans with Sesame Hummus

Ready in Time: 10 minutes | Servings: 6

Ingredients

4 Tbsp sesame oil

2 cloves garlic finely sliced

1 can (15 oz) cannellini beans, drained 4 Tbsp sesame paste

2 Tbsp lemon juice freshly squeezed 1/4 tsp red pepper flakes

2 Tbsp fresh basil finely chopped

2 Tbsp fresh parsley finely choppedSea salt to taste

Instructions

1. Place all ingredients in your food processor.

2. Process until all ingredients are combined well and smooth.

3. Transfer mixture into a bowl and refrigerate until

servings.

Nutrition Facts

Percent daily values based on the Reference Daily Intake (RDI) for a2000 calorie diet.

Amount Per Serving

Calories 491.59 | Calories From Fat (74%) 365.15 | Total Fat 43.14g 66%

| Saturated Fat 6.09g 30% |

Cholesterol 0mg 0% | Sodium 108.39mg 5% | Potassium 521.26mg 15% | Total Carbohydrates 20.71g 7% | Fiber 6g 23% | Sugar 0.73g | Protein 13.33g 27%

33. Candied Honey-Coconut Peanuts

Ready in Time: 15 minutes | Servings: 8

Ingredients

1/2 cup honey (preferably a darker honey) 4 Tbsp coconut butter softened

1 tsp ground cinnamon

4 cups roasted, salted peanuts

Instructions

1. Add honey, coconut butter, and cinnamon in a microwave-safebowl.

2. Microwave at HIGH for about 4 to 5 minutes.

3. Stir in nuts; mix thoroughly to coat.

4. Microwave at HIGH 5 to 6 minutes or until foamy; stir after 3minutes.

5. Spread in a single layer on a greased tray.

6. Refrigerated for 6 hours.

7. Break into small pieces and serve.

Nutrition Facts

Percent daily values based on the Reference Daily Intake (RDI) for a2000 calorie diet.

Amount Per Serving

Calories 550.88 | Calories From Fat (66%) 361.89 | Total Fat 43g 66% | Saturated Fat 10.92g 55% |

Cholesterol 0mg 0% | Sodium 5.26mg <1% | Potassium 492.76mg 14% | Total Carbohydrates 33.42g 11% | Fiber 6g 24% | Sugar 20.46g | Protein 17.36g 35%

34.   **Choco Walnuts Fat Bombs**

Preparation Time: 15 minutes | Servings: 6

Ingredients

1/2 cup coconut butter

1/2 cup coconut oil softened

4 Tbs cocoa powder, unsweetened 4 Tbs brown sugar firmly packed 1/3 cup silken tofu mashed

1 cup walnuts, roughly chopped

Instructions

1.   Add coconut butter and coconut oil into a microwave dish; meltit for 10-15 seconds.

2. Add in cocoa powder and whisk well.

3.   Pour mixture into a blender with brown sugar and silken tofucream; blend for 3-4 minutes.

4. Place silicone molds onto a sheet pan and fill halfway with choppedwalnuts.

5. Pour the mixture over the walnuts and place it in the freezer for 6hours.

6. Ready! Serve!

Nutrition Facts

Percent daily values based on the Reference Daily Intake (RDI) for a2000 calorie diet.

Amount Per Serving

Calories 506 | Calories From Fat (86%) 435.7 | Total Fat 50.44g 78% |Saturated Fat 28.16g 141% |

Cholesterol 0mg 0% | Sodium 5.38mg <1% | Potassium 213mg 6% |Total Carbohydrates 14.72g 5% |

Fiber 2.54g 10% | Sugar 9g | Protein 5.29g 11%

35.   **Crispy Honey Pecans (Slow Cooker)**

Ready in Time: 2 hours and 15 minutes | Servings: 4

Ingredients

16 oz pecan halves

4 Tbsp coconut butter melted 4 to 5 Tbsp honey strained 1/4 tsp ground ginger

1/4 tsp ground allspice

1 1/2 tsp ground cinnamon

Instructions

1.   Add pecans and melted coconut butter into your 4-quart SlowCooker.

2. Stir until combined well.

3. Add in honey and stir well.

4. In a bowl, combine spices and sprinkle over nuts; stir lightly.

5. Cook on LOW uncovered for about 2 to 3 hours or until nuts arecrispy.

6. Serve cold.

Nutrition Facts

Percent daily values based on the Reference Daily Intake (RDI) for a2000 calorie diet.

Amount Per Serving

Calories 852 | Calories From Fat (82%) 784.5 | Total Fat 93.15g 143% | Saturated Fat 14,31g 72% |

Cholesterol 30.53mg 10% | Sodium 2.61mg <1% | Potassium 485.23mg 14% | Total Carbohydrates 33.2g 11% | Fiber 11.47g 46% | Sugar 21.78g | Protein 10.63g 21%

36.   **Crunchy Fried Pickles**

Ready in Time: 5 minutes | Servings: 6

Ingredients

1/2 cup Vegetable oil for frying1 cup all-purpose flour

1 cup plain breadcrumbsPinch of salt and pepper

30 pickle chips (cucumber, dill)

Instructions

1. Heat oil in a large frying skillet over medium-high heat.

2.   Stir the flour, breadcrumbs, and the salt and pepper in a shallowbowl.

3.   Dredge   the   pickles   in   the flour/breadcrumbs mixture to coatcompletely.

4. Fry in batches until golden brown on all sides, 2 to 3 minutes in total.

5. Drain on paper towels and serve.

Nutrition Facts

Percent daily values based on the Reference Daily Intake (RDI) for a2000 calorie diet.

Amount Per Serving

Calories 328.53 | Calories From Fat (53%) 172.76 | Total Fat 19.57g 30%

| Saturated Fat 1.65g 8% |

Cholesterol 0mg 0% | Sodium 1063.43mg 49% | Potassium 218.57mg 6% | Total Carbohydrates 33.39g 11% | Fiber 3.3g 13% | Sugar 3.46g | Protein 5.61g 11%

37. Banana and Peanut Butter Tortillas

Ready in Time: 15 minutes | Servings: 4

Ingredients

1/3 cup peanut butter

4 medium tortillas

2 large bananas sliced 3 Tbsp peanut oil Pinch of Kosher salt

Pine Honey for serving (optional)

Instructions

1. Heat a non-stick frying skillet over medium heat.

2. Spread peanut butter over the tortilla.

3. Over half of tortilla arrange the banana slices, sprinkle with a pinch of salt, and top with the remaining tortilla, peanut butter side down.

4. Stick them together and then brush both sides lightly with peanut oil.

5. Place each tortilla in a hot frying pan and cook, flipping once, forabout 2 minutes per side.

6. When ready, remove tortillas onto a plate and let cool

completely.

7. Cut each tortilla into quarters; store in an airtight container and keeprefrigerated up to 5 days.

Nutrition Facts

Percent daily values based on the Reference Daily Intake (RDI) for a2000 calorie diet.

Amount Per Serving

Calories 371.59 | Calories From Fat (56%) 206.9 | Total Fat 24g 37% | Saturated Fat 3.7g 19% | Cholesterol 0mg 0% | Sodium 302.79mg 13% | Potassium 400.35mg 11% | Total Carbohydrates 34.11g 11% | Fiber 3.82g 15% | Sugar 9.81g | Protein 8.69g 18%

38.   Barbecue Bean Dip (Instant Pot)

Ready in Time: 20 minutes | Servings: 8

Ingredients

1 can (15 oz) cannellini beans rinsed

1   can (6 oz) red beans rinsed and drained 1/2 cup onion finely diced

2   cloves garlic minced 4 Tbsp Barbecue sauce 1/2 cup tomato sauce

3/4 cup vegan ricotta or vegan brie 1 Tbsp fresh parsley chopped table salt to taste

Instructions

1. Add all ingredients in your Instant Pot.

2. Lock lid into place and set on the MANUAL setting for 15 minutes.

   3. When the timer beeps, press "Cancel" and carefully flip the Quick Release valve to let the pressure out.

4. Using an immersion blender, blend the mixture until soft.

5. Transfer dip into the container, and allow to cool down completely.

6. Keep refrigerated up to 5 days.

Nutrition Facts

Percent daily values based on the Reference Daily Intake (RDI) for a 2000 calorie diet.

Amount Per Serving

Calories 297.81 | Calories From Fat (7%) 21.84 | Total Fat 2.5g 4% | Saturated Fat 0.42g 2% | Cholesterol 0mg 0% | Sodium 233.63mg 10% | Potassium 1410.7mg 40% | Total Carbohydrates 50.69g 17% | Fiber 12.19g 49% | Sugar 3.7g | Protein 20.23g 40%

39. **Breaded Cauliflower Florets**

Ready in Time: 45 minutes | Servings: 6

Ingredients

1 large head of cauliflower

1 cup rice flour (besan or wheat flour)1 tsp salt

3/4 tsp garlic powder3/4 cup water

1 cup chili sauce

2 Tbsp plant butter (any) softened

Instructions

1. Preheat oven to 420 F.

2. Line a large baking sheet with parchment paper; set aside.

3. Rise, clean and cut cauliflower into florets; place in a large bowl.

4. In a separate bowl, combine the rice flour, salt, garlic powder, andwater; stir well.

5. Pour the mixture evenly over the cauliflower florets and toss tocombine well.

6. Place cauliflower on a prepared baking sheet in a single layer.

7. Place in oven and bake for 15 minutes.

8. In a bowl, whisk together hot sauce and vegetable butter.

9. Transfer the cauliflower to a large bowl.

10. Pour the sauce evenly over cauliflower pieces.

11. Transfer the cauliflower back on the baking sheet and for further 15minutes.

12. Remove the cauliflower from the oven and set aside to cool down.

13. Refrigerate the cauliflower in an airtight container up to 4 days.

Nutrition Facts

Percent daily values based on the Reference Daily Intake (RDI) for a 2000 calorie diet.

Amount Per Serving

Calories 98.51 | Calories From Fat (29%) 28.58 | Total Fat 3.41g 5% | Saturated Fat 0.31g 2% | Cholesterol 0mg 0% | Sodium 732.57mg 31% | Potassium 375.9mg 11% | Total Carbohydrates 14.43g 5% | Fiber 2.88g 12% | Sugar 2.4g | Protein 4.24g 8%

40. **Coconut- Berry Cream with Turmeric**

Ready in Time: 10 minutes | Servings: 4

Ingredients

1 1/2 cups coconut milk canned 1 Tbsp coconut cream softened

1 cup of frozen berries (blueberries, bilberries, raspberries) 1 cup fresh pineapple cut into pieces

1 small banana sliced (frozen or fresh) 1/2 tsp turmeric, freshly grated

2 to 3 Tbsp coconut palm sugar (or granulated sugar)

Instructions

1. Place all ingredients in your fast-speed blender.

2. Blend until smooth and combined well.

3. Taste and adjust sugar to taste.

4. Keep refrigerated in a glass container or jar for up to 5 days.

Nutrition Facts

Percent daily values based on the Reference Daily Intake (RDI) for a 2000 calorie diet.

Amount Per Serving

Calories 252.46 | Calories From Fat (61%) 154.42 | Total Fat 18.5g 28% | Saturated Fat 16.16g 81% | Cholesterol 0mg 0% | Sodium 12.17mg <1% | Potassium 358mg 10% | Total Carbohydrates 24.32g 8% | Fiber 2.19g 9% | Sugar 14.42g | Protein 2.51g 5%

41.   **Creamy Eggplant-Flax Dip**

Ready in Time: 20 minutes | Servings: 10

Ingredients

2 eggplants peeled and cut into pieces 1 small onion chopped into small dices3 Tbsp olive oil

2 clove garlic minced or mashed 1/3 cup of flaxseed flour

1 cup vegetable broth

salt and ground black pepper t to taste 1 cup of vegan mayonnaise

Instructions

1. Peel, rinse and cut eggplant lengthwise into pieces.

2. Add all ingredients (except Mayo) in your Instant Pot; give a good stir.

    3. Lock lid into place and set on the MANUAL setting high pressure for10 minutes.

    4. When the beep sounds, quick release the pressure by pressing Cancel, and twisting the steam handle to the Venting position.

5. Remove the mixture into your blender or food

processor.

6. Add vegan mayonnaise, and season with the salt and pepper; stir untilsmooth and creamy.

7. Allow to cool completely, and keep refrigerated in a sealed containerup to 5 days.

Nutrition Facts

Percent daily values based on the Reference Daily Intake (RDI) for a2000 calorie diet.

Amount Per Serving

Calories 223.81 | Calories From Fat (83%) 184.79 | Total Fat 19g 29%

| Saturated Fat 1.48g 7% | Cholesterol 0.25mg <1%

| Sodium 277.11mg 12% | Potassium 269.6mg 8% |

Total Carbohydrates 9.19g 3% | Fiber 3.65g 15% |

Sugar 2.68g | Protein 1.69g 3%

SWEETS/DESSERTS

42.   Sunrise Peach Marmalade

Servings: 4

Ingredients

4 cups fresh peaches diced1/2 cup peach juice

1 Tbsp finely grated orange peel 3 Tbsp honey extracted

1 Tbsp lemon juice

Instructions

1.   Place all ingredients in a blender or food processor; blend untilcombined well.

2. Pour mixture into a glass microwave-safe dish.

3. Uncovered, microwave on HIGH for 15 to 17 minutes, stirring every 5minutes.

4. Allow it to cool.

5. Serve with crusty bread, ice cream, fruits...etc.

6. Keep refrigerated.

Nutrition Facts

Percent daily values based on the Reference Daily Intake (RDI) for a2000 calorie diet.

Amount Per Serving

Calories 130.22 | Calories From Fat (3%) 3.69 | Total Fat 0.5g <1% |Saturated Fat 0,04g <1% |

Cholesterol 0mg 0% | Sodium 2mg <1% | Potassium 378.3mg 11% |Total Carbohydrates 33.5g 11% |

Fiber 3.16g 13% | Sugar 30.5g | Protein 2g 4%

43.   **Vegan Blueberry Ice Cream**

Preparation Time: 20 minutes | Servings: 8

Ingredients

4 cups fresh blueberries (or frozen blueberries)1 1/2 cups granulated sugar

2 Tbsp water

1 Tbsp arrowroot powder

2 cups coconut cream softened

Instructions

1. Add blueberries, sugar, and water in a saucepan.

2. Cook, frequently stirring, over medium heat; bring to a boil.

3. Reduce heat to low and stir for about 10 minutes over low heat or untilblueberries are softened,

4. Strain the mixture, and discard seeds and skins.

5. Add the coconut cream and beat with an electric mixer until soft andcreamy.

6. Pour the mixture in a freezer-safe container and freeze for 4 to 5 hours.

7. Transfer frozen mixture to a bowl and

beat with a mixer until smooth to avoid ice cream crystallization.

8. Repeat this process at least 4 times.

9. Remove from the freezer 15 minutes before servings.

Nutrition Facts

Percent daily values based on the Reference Daily Intake (RDI) for a2000 calorie diet.

Amount Per Serving

Calories 242.9 | Calories From Fat (70%) 170.2 | Total Fat 21.05g 32% |Saturated Fat 18.47g 92% |

Cholesterol 0mg 0% | Sodium 3.26mg <1% | Potassium 250.7mg 7% | Total Carbohydrates 17.25g 6% | Fiber 3g 12% | Sugar 7.22g | Protein 2.72g 5%

44. Vegan Hazelnut - Coffee Truffles

Preparation Time: 25 minutes | Servings: 12

Ingredients

Base:

1   1/2 cups hazelnuts (soaked)1/4 cup water

1/4 cup maple syrupPinch of sea salt

2 tsp vanilla seeds

1 Tbsp coffee extract

1/4 cup coconut oil softenedGlaze:

1/2 cup coconut oil softened1/2 cup cacao powder

1/4 cup maple syrupa pinch of salt

Instructions

1. Add all base ingredients into a food processor; process until smoothand well incorporated.

2. Pour mixture into a bowl and place in the freezer until firm.

3. Shape mixture into balls (about 12).

4. Place on foil and place back in the freezer to harden.

5. To make a glaze: whisk together all glaze ingredients until smooth.

6. Dip balls into the glaze mixture and place them on the foil.

7. Place them back in the freezer to set completely.

Nutrition Facts

Percent daily values based on the Reference Daily Intake (RDI) for a2000 calorie diet.

Amount Per Serving

Calories 297.45 | Calories From Fat (77%) 230.4 | Total Fat 27.12g 42% |Saturated Fat 13g 65% |

Cholesterol 0mg 0% | Sodium 2.57mg <1% | Potassium 241.38mg 7% | Total Carbohydrates 14.68g 5% | Fiber 3.15g 13% | Sugar 9.15g | Protein 3.84g 8%

45. Vegan Protein - Chocolate Ice Cream

Preparation Time: 20 minutes | Servings: 5

Ingredients

1 can (15 oz) coconut milk, unsweetened 1 Tbsp cornflour

1/4 cup cacao powder, unsweetened 1/4 cup maple syrup

1 tsp vanilla extract

2 scoop protein powder (pea or soy)

For serving/garnish - chopped walnuts and golden raisins

Instructions

1. Combine together all ingredients into a high-speed blender and blend until creamy and smooth.

2. Transfer the mixture in a freezer-safe container and freeze until firm(not less than 4 hours).

3. Transfer frozen mixture to a bowl and

beat with a mixer to break up the ice crystals. Repeat this process at least 4 times.

4. Let the ice cream at room temperature for 15 minutes before serving.

Nutrition Facts

Percent daily values based on the Reference Daily Intake (RDI) for a2000 calorie diet.

Amount Per Serving

Calories 358.78 | Calories From Fat (72%) 259.5 | Total Fat 31g 48% | Saturated Fat 17.59g 88% |

Cholesterol 0.92mg <1% | Sodium 28.2mg 1% | Potassium 418mg 12% | Total Carbohydrates 19.85g 7% | Fiber 3g 12% | Sugar 10.43g | Protein 8g 16%

46.   **Winter Pumpkin Pancakes**

Ready in Time: S0 minutes | Servings: 6

Ingredients

2 cups all-purpose flour

2 Tbsp brown sugar - (packed)1 Tbsp baking powder

1 1/4 tsp pumpkin pie spicePinch or two of salt

1 3/4 cups almond milk

1/2 cup pure pumpkin (canned) 1 Tbsp silken tofu mashed

2   Tbsp sesame oilServing

Honey

Chopped nuts (optional)

Instructions

1. In a large bowl, combine together flour, brown sugar, baking powder,pumpkin pie spice, and salt.

2. In a separate bowl, stir almond milk, pumpkin, silken tofu, and sesameoil.

3. Add almond milk mixture to the flour mixture; stir just untilmoistened.

4. Heat griddle or skillet over medium heat; brush lightly with vegetableoil.

5. Pour 1/4 cup batter onto hot griddle; cook until bubbles begin to burst.

6. Turn and continue cooking 1 to 2 minutes. Repeat with the remainingbatter.

7. Serve with hot with honey and chopped nuts.

Nutrition Facts

Percent daily values based on the Reference Daily Intake (RDI) for a2000 calorie diet.

Amount Per Serving

Calories 295.39 | Calories From Fat (36%) 105.84 | Total Fat 12.33g 19%

| Saturated Fat 1.32g 7% |

Cholesterol 31mg 10% | Sodium 694.91mg 29% | Potassium 150.12mg 4% | Total Carbohydrates 40.22g 13% | Fiber 2.43g 10% | Sugar 5.45g | Protein 7.7g 16%

47. Rugged" Coconut Balls

Ready in Time: 15 minutes | Servings: 8

Ingredients

1/3 cup coconut oil melted

1/3 cup coconut butter softened

1 oz coconut, finely shredded, unsweetened 4 Tbsp coconut palm sugar

1/2 cup shredded coconut

Instructions

1. Combine all ingredients in a blender.

2. Blend until soft and well combined.

3. Form small balls from the mixture and roll in shredded coconut.

4. Place on a sheet lined with parchment paper and refrigerate overnight.

5. Keep coconut balls into sealed container in fridge up to one week.

Nutrition Facts

Percent daily values based on the Reference Daily Intake (RDI) for a 2000 calorie diet.

Amount Per Serving

Calories 226.89 | Calories From Fat (84%) 190.39 |
Total Fat 21.6g 34% | Saturated Fat 19.84g 99% |
Cholesterol 0mg 0% | Sodium 17.19mg <1% |

Potassium 45mg 1% | Total Carbohydrates 9g 3% |
Fiber 1.16g 5% | Sugar5.7g | Protein 1g 2%

48. **Almond - Choco Cake**

Ready in Time: 45 minutes | Servings: 8

Ingredients

1 1/2 cups of almond flour

1/3 cup almonds finely chopped

1/4 cup of cocoa powder unsweetenedPinch of salt

1/2 tsp baking soda 2 Tbsp almond milk

1/2 cup Coconut oil melted2 tsp pure vanilla extract

1/3 cup brown sugar (packed)

Instructions

1. Preheat oven to 350 F.

2. Line 9" cake pan with parchment paper, and grease with a little meltedcoconut oil; set aside.

3. Stir the almond flour, chopped almonds, cocoa powder, salt, andbaking soda in a bowl.

4. In a separate bowl, stir the remaining ingredients.

5. Combine the almond flour mixture with the almond milk mixture andstir well.

6. Place batter in a prepared cake pan.

7. Bake for 30 to 32 minutes.

8. Remove from the oven, allow it to cool completely.

9. Store the cake-slices a freezer, tightly wrapped in a double layer ofplastic wrap and a layer of foil. It will keep on this way for up to a month.

Nutrition Facts

Percent daily values based on the Reference Daily Intake (RDI) for a 2000 calorie diet.

Amount Per Serving

Calories 195.61 | Calories From Fat (74%) 145.59 | Total Fat 16.9g 26% | Saturated Fat 12.23g 61% | Cholesterol 0mg 0% | Sodium 118.39mg 5% | Potassium 95.64mg 3% | Total Carbohydrates 11.9g 4% | Fiber 1.52g 6% | Sugar 9.35g | Protein 1.75g 4%

49.   **Banana-Almond Cake**

Ready in Time: 1 hour | Servings: 8

Ingredients

4 ripe bananas in chunks

3 Tbsš honey or maple syrup 1 tsp pure vanilla extract

1/2 cup almond milk

3/4 cup of self-raising flour 1 tsp cinnamon

1 tsp baking powder 1 pinch of salt

1/3 cup of almonds finely chopped Almond slices for decoration

Instructions

1. Preheat the oven to 400 F (air mode).

2. Oil a cake mold; set aside.

3. Add bananas into a bowl and mash with the fork.

4. Add honey, vanilla, almond, and stir well.

5. In a separate bowl, stir flour, cinnamon, baking powder, salt, the almonds broken, and mix with a spoon.

6. Combine the flour mixture with the banana mixture, and stir until allingredients combined well.

7. Transfer the mixture to prepared cake mold and sprinkle with slicedalmonds.

8. Bake for 40-45 minutes or until the toothpick inserted comes out clean.

9. Remove from the oven, and allow the cake to cool completely.

10. Cut cake into slices, place in tin foil, or an airtight container, and keep refrigerated up to one week.

Nutrition Facts

Percent daily values based on the Reference Daily Intake (RDI) for a2000 calorie diet.

Amount Per Serving

Calories 155.94 | Calories From Fat (18%) 27.68 | Total Fat 3.31g 5% | Saturated Fat 0.32g 2% | Cholesterol 0mg 0% | Sodium 98.68mg 4% | Potassium 271mg 8% | Total Carbohydrates 30.61g 10% | Fiber 2.67g 11% |Sugar 14g | Protein 3.6g 7%

50.   **Banana-Coconut Ice Cream**

Ready in Time: 15 minutes | Servings: 6

Ingredients

1   cup coconut cream 1/2 cup Inverted sugar

2   large frozen bananas (chunks) 3 Tbsp honey extracted

1/4 tsp cinnamon powder

Instructions

1. In a bowl, whip the coconut cream with the inverted sugar.

2. In a separate bowl, beat the banana with honey and cinnamon.

3. Incorporate the coconut whipped cream and banana mixture; stir well.

4. Cover the bowl and let cool in the refrigerator over the night.

5. Stir the mixture 3 to 4 times to avoid crystallization.

6. Keep frozen 1 to 2 months.

Nutrition Facts

Percent daily values based on the Reference

Daily Intake (RDI) for a2000 calorie diet.

Amount Per Serving

Calories 253 | Calories From Fat (46%) 117.23 | Total Fat 14g 22% | Saturated Fat 12.35g 62% | Cholesterol 0mg 0% | Sodium 2.45mg <1% | Potassium 275.25mg 8% | Total Carbohydrates 34.16g 11% | Fiber 1.97g 8% | Sugar 27.19g | Protein 1.91g 4%

CPSIA information can be obtained
at www.ICGtesting.com
Printed in the USA
LVHW081656230521
688193LV00024B/405